Food Allergies

Merri Lou Dobler, MS, RD

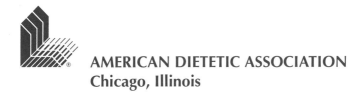

AMERICAN DIETETIC ASSOCIATION
Chicago, Illinois

10 9 8 7 6 5 4

Contents

Introduction

Do you avoid certain foods because you "react" to them? Do you wonder if you or your child have food allergies? Are you confused about tests for food allergy diagnosis? Answers to your questions and concerns are addressed in this booklet on food allergies from the American Dietetic Association. *Food Allergies* includes the following information:

- Symptoms, Medical Intervention
- Nutrition Highlights, Meal Planning
- Label Reading
- Resources, References
- Special Products
- Recipes

The topic of food allergies and adverse reactions to food is controversial, even among members of the medical profession. Physical symptoms are often associated with food. The incidence of true food allergy has been estimated to range from 0.3% to 7% among children in the United States, with allergic reactions to many foods, such as milk, decreasing with age. Some allergic reactions, however, are so severe that in many cases even the smell of or skin contact with offending foods, such as peanuts and shrimp, can cause mild or even severe physical responses.

Many people claim they have "food allergies." A wide variety of terms more clearly define reactions to foods. Don't let the terms "food allergy," "food intolerance," and "food sensitivity" confuse you. Health professionals use definitions adopted by the American Academy of Allergy and Immunology Committee on Adverse Reactions to Foods. You will find simplified definitions helpful:

Adverse reaction to food: Any abnormal reaction to a food or food additive.

Allergic reaction to food or food hypersensitivity: A reaction of the immune system as a result of eating a food. A true food allergy can be tested clinically because of changes in the immune system.

Food intolerance: A reaction to a food or food additive that is not caused by a reaction in the immune system. This is a nonallergic reaction to a food or food additive. The symptoms may be very similar to an allergic reaction. A food intolerance such as lactose intolerance (see the American Dietetic Association's *Lactose Intolerance*) is due to a deficiency in the intestines of the digestive enzyme lactase.

Reactions to food may occur because natural substances in certain foods, such as mushrooms or rhubarb, can be toxic to the body. Contaminants of food, such as molds in peanuts or corn or pesticides in foods, may cause adverse reactions when large amounts of the food are consumed.

A true food allergy can be clinically tested because of immune system changes. Antibodies are an immune system response. Antibodies develop when the offending food protein, which is known as an *allergen*, is consumed. Large amounts of antibodies, which are measured in the body as "immunoglobulins," may develop after you eat a certain food, or food allergen, such as walnuts. It is the measurement of these antibodies, or immunoglobulins, and the adverse physical symptoms you experience when you consume a food allergen that determines a true food allergy or food hypersensitivity.

Many people are familiar with allergy medications called antihistamines. These medicines are available by prescription or over the counter (OTC) and they block the development of histamines in the body. *Histamines* are body chemicals produced when an allergic reaction takes place in the body. Histamines cause many reactions, especially skin reactions, such as hives, and runny nose.

Please Note!

This dietary information is not a substitute for medical diagnosis and supervision of food allergy management. Contact your physician for consultation and a registered dietitian (RD) for nutrition information.

Symptoms

Reactions to foods usually occur in a period ranging from within seconds to up to 2 hours after eating a food. However, reactions may be delayed for 1 to 2 days and produce more subtle results. Some of the foods that typically result in physical symptoms include milk, nuts, egg, soy, peas, fish, and shellfish such as shrimp. Foods such as soy, milk, wheat, and egg produce food allergies that are frequently outgrown, whereas allergies produced by peanuts, nuts, fish, and shellfish are less commonly outgrown. The food or foods that trigger a reaction vary with the individual, and no one can predict whether he or she will be allergic to a food just because that food is commonly noted to cause reactions.

There are different types of physical responses to allergic substances. These symptoms, it should be noted, may also be due to other causes. Medical evaluation is necessary for diagnosis of allergic responses due to food.

Skin Reactions

- Swelling of the lips, mouth, tongue, face, or throat
- Hives
- Rashes

Nose, Throat, and Lung Reactions

- Sneezes
- Nasal congestion
- Chronic coughs
- Asthma

Stomach and Intestinal Reactions

- Nausea
- Abdominal pain and bloating
- Vomiting
- Diarrhea
- Cramping
- Gas

Anaphylactic Reactions

An anaphylactic reaction is a whole-body systemic reaction to a food. Body responses may include any combination of skin reactions; nose, throat, and lung reactions; and stomach and intestinal reactions. Many reactions at the same time can overwhelm an individual. Anaphylactic reactions can occur in a few seconds or minutes, with symptoms that include nausea, diarrhea, chest pain and heart arrhythmias, hives, asthma, low blood pressure, and shock. Immediate action by an alert and knowledgeable individual can prevent serious results. Without immediate medical attention, death may result. Foods implicated in anaphylactic reactions include peanuts and tree nuts, eggs, and shellfish.

Controversial Reactions

Physical symptoms such as recurrent ear infections, arthritis, migraine headaches, urinary tract infections, behavioral problems, and hyperactivity have not been definitively linked to food allergies and may have other causes. The relationship between food allergy and these areas are topics of continuing research. Contact your local medical society or physician referral source for medical assistance and treatment of these problems.

Medical Intervention

Your physician will review your medical and diet history and conduct a thorough physical exam. Diagnostic tests such as skin and blood testing may be recommended to detect the presence of antibodies and the probability of allergic reactions.

Skin Testing

Two skin tests, the scratch test and the puncture or prick skin test, use extracts of foods that are injected under the skin to detect the presence of allergic antibodies to specific foods. Approximately 15 to 20 minutes after the application of extracts, the punctured area is examined for a *wheal and flare*, a round bump or mosquito bite-like response on the skin indicating a reaction. A reaction indicates the possibility of antibodies and the resulting release of histamine. Skin reactions, however, do not always correlate with responses after eating foods and are a topic of continuing debate in the medical community. Negative reactions to skin tests indicate a high probability of no sensitivity.

RAST

Another appropriate test helpful in diagnosing food allergy is the radioallergosorbent test (RAST), which uses a blood sample. This expensive test can be incorrectly interpreted. Make sure it is done by a board-certified allergist or physician.

Food Challenges

Open challenges, single blind challenges, and double blind placebo-controlled food challenges (DBPCFC), conducted under physician supervision, are also used for diagnosis. The most accurate food challenge test for food allergy diagnosis is the DBPCFC, designed to control for subjectivity by the patient and physician. After a week to 10 days on an elimination diet, which allows the person to eat foods that will not produce reactions and will reduce current physical symptoms, the individual is given an opaque capsule to swallow. The capsule contains either the offending food substance in powder form or a powdered substance that is known not to cause reactions. Neither the physician nor the individual is aware which substance is being administered. In the absence of symptoms, the powdered food may be given in increasingly larger doses, and all symptoms are recorded.

Intestinal Biopsy

A biopsy of the small intestine is often used for diagnosis of abnormalities of the intestinal tract, such as celiac disease, which requires a gluten-free diet (see the American Dietetic Association's *Gluten Intolerance)*. White blood cell counts and nasal smears of certain cells called *eosinophils* in conjunction with other tests are also used to ascertain food allergies.

Controversial tests and treatment for food allergies include sublingual food drops, cytotoxic food testing, food injections, and certain dietary elimination diets, such as the Feingold diet. Consult with your allergist or physician for more information on these tests.

Nutrition Highlights

Diets That Help in Diagnosing Food Allergies

The best treatment for food allergy is elimination of the offending food from your diet. If whole groups of foods are dropped from your diet, you may miss essential vitamins and minerals. Essential nutrients contributed from cow's milk, for instance, include calcium, vitamins A and D, riboflavin, and protein. Do not assume that vitamin-mineral supplements can take the place of a diet lacking in essential nutrients; check with a registered dietitian (RD) for nutritionally adequate foods to substitute for foods you are avoiding.

Food diary—A food diary is an in-depth record of foods, beverages, and medications consumed, in addition to any symptoms experienced, usually in a 2-to-4-week time period. It is used to help pinpoint foods and groups of foods that may cause you physical discomfort and to determine the nutritional adequacy of the diet.

Elimination diet—An elimination diet is designed as a short-term modification to your diet to reduce physical symptoms and determine offending foods. Elimination diets are composed of limited numbers of foods that you can eat and other foods that you must avoid. Rice, lamb, sweet potatoes, and carrots are examples of foods generally allowed on an elimination diet. These diets are often or usually not nutritionally complete. They require assistance in planning so that they may be successfully completed, and they should be temporary.

An improvement in physical symptoms is one step in determining dietary problems. The elimination diet then is followed by the careful reintroduction of suspected foods in a sequential format and the observation of symptoms. An elimination diet includes keeping a food diary to record food intake and symptoms. The final goal is an adequate diet with as few restricted foods as possible.

Food challenges—Food challenges may be used to confirm results of skin tests. Only foods confirmed by a food challenge should remain prohibited, and these may be challenged at specified intervals, for example, every 6 months. When there is a severe reaction to foods, however, challenges *must* be done *only* under direct medical supervision with emergency services available. Minute amounts of foods are given, followed by larger amounts at specified time intervals. All reactions are noted.

Meal Planning

The basis of food allergy management is a knowledgeable consumer with supermarket savvy, restaurant know-how, and a lot of patience. When a physician recommends an elimination diet, periodic food challenges, or a food diary, an RD can provide assistance and instructions in successfully carrying these out.

A guideline for meal planning for the food allergic individual is based on the Food Guide Pyramid, found in the USDA's *Dietary Guidelines for Americans,* 4th ed, 1995, Home and Garden Bulletin No 232. For good health, eat a variety of foods and select *at least* the lower number of servings below. There are many types of food in all food groups except milk so the allergic individual has many options.

Food Group	Suggested No. of Servings	Serving Size
Vegetables	3–5	1 cup raw leafy or ½ cup cooked
Fruits	2–4	1 medium size or ½ cup canned or ¾ cup juice
Grain products (breads, cereals, rice, and pasta)	6–11	1 slice bread or 1 ounce ready-to-eat cereal or ½ cup cooked cereal, rice, or pasta
Milk (milk, yogurt, cheese, and equivalents)	2–3	1 cup milk/yogurt or 1½ oz cheese or 2 ounces processed cheese
Meat and beans (meats, poultry, fish, dry beans and peas, eggs, and nuts)	2–3	2-3 oz cooked or ½ cup cooked beans or 1 egg or 2 tablespoons peanut butter or ⅓ cup nuts
Fats, oils, and sweets	Use sparingly	
Alcohol	Use in moderation	

Concerns about Infants

Infants with food allergies may develop eczema and diarrhea and later exhibit symptoms of asthma and allergic rhinitis, or "hay fever," as they grow older. Some cases of colic have been associated with food allergies.

Bloody diarrhea and failure to thrive in infants are often linked to cow's milk allergy. For infants with a family history of allergies, who are therefore at risk of developing allergies, exclusive breast-feeding for the first 6 to 12 months may delay the appearance of allergic symptoms. Breast-feeding will probably not completely prevent allergies in children who are at high risk of developing allergies. A nutritionally complete diet is strongly recommended for pregnant women with allergies, as for all women.

New Skills

An RD is knowledgeable in food allergy management and can help you learn necessary management and coping skills. Ingredient substitution becomes second nature with a little practice and a lot of kitchen experimentation. Your blender, food processor, and mixer can be invaluable helpers. Seek advice on local stores that carry specialty items. Extra time will be needed to prepare foods and plan menus, especially at first.

Brown-bag your lunch if you are unsure what food will be served when eating out. Offer to bring food you can enjoy to parties. Choose restaurants carefully; check beforehand with restaurant personnel regarding menu items, and ask lots of questions. Choose plain foods if in doubt about food ingredients.

Label Reading

Label reading is an important skill for the food-allergic individual. Food manufacturers may change ingredients and labels without warning, which keeps you on your toes checking labels. Ambiguous wording on labels is a warning sign, especially for the very sensitive person who must avoid all contact with certain foods. Contact companies for specific ingredient information and refer to publications that provide lists of food ingredients (see "Resources," "References," and "Special Products"). Check larger supermarkets, health food stores, and Oriental and specialty food stores for alternatives.

Cow's Milk

Cow's milk allergy is believed to be the most common food allergy experienced among food allergic individuals. It may be seen in up to 30% of children with allergies and 2% to 7.5% of all infants. Check food labels and products for the following words, which indicate the presence of cow's milk. You may tolerate some milk-containing foods and should check with your physician and RD before eliminating all sources of cow's milk from your diet.

butter	nonfat milk solids	chocolate (products may use milk solids)
milk	whey	
yogurt	ghee	casein
cheese	cream	sodium caseinate
cottage cheese	ice cream	lactoglobulin
curds	buttermilk	lactalbumin

Substitutions and Dietary Management

Foods that typically contain milk include many baked products, such as cakes, doughnuts, and breads, salad dressings, frozen desserts, creamed foods and soups, and processed lunch meats. Check labels on egg substitutes, gravy mixes, and diet beverages.

Alternatives

Alternatives to milk-containing products include soy, rice, almond, oat and grain liquid beverages, imitation cheeses and soybean curd (tofu). Tofu-based products are excellent substitutes for comparable milk-containing products. Some cocoa products do not contain milk solids. Kosher foods are often milk-free and will say "pareve" or "parve" on the label, but the label must be read to confirm this. Milk-free margarines are available.

Other fluids substitute very well in recipes. Apple juice, for instance, is an acceptable substitution in pancakes. Water, fruit juices, soy milk, and broths can add variety.

Infant Formulas

A variety of soybean formulas, "predigested" formulas, and meat-based formulas for infants are available (see "Special Products" or contact an RD for more information).

Nondairy Foods

Inadequate substitutes for cow's milk are nondairy creamers, which do not contain high-quality protein or calcium and are lower in vitamins and minerals than milk. Check labels of nondairy foods in the refrigerated or freezer section of your supermarket for the addition of milk. The fat substitute Simplesse, which is used in frozen dairy products, contains milk protein and should be avoided.

Wheat

Check food labels and grain products for the following ingredients, which contain wheat protein. You may tolerate some wheat products and should check with your physician and RD before eliminating all sources of wheat from your diet.

wheat	all-purpose flour	graham flour
wheat germ	pastry flour	farina
semolina	cake flour	modified food starch
graham	gluten flour	malt or cereal extract
bran		

Substitutions and Dietary Management

Foods that contain wheat include many baked products, such as breads and desserts, crackers, gravy, pancake mixes, and cereals. Avoid products that use wheat as a filler, such as bologna and luncheon meats. Salad dressings may be thickened with wheat flour, and breaded products may contain wheat. Alcoholic beverages such as beer may contain wheat.

Alternatives

Nonwheat starchy foods for mealtime include potatoes, rice, rice and corn cakes, corn or rice noodles, and mung beans (Chinese bean threads). Rice cereals and flaked corn cereals or cornmeal can be used for breading foods. Some packaged cold-cereal products are specifically designed for the wheat-allergic and gluten-intolerant person.

Flour Substitutions

Alternative flours for cooking and baking include barley, buckwheat, oat, rye, rice, potato starch, and soy flour. Substitutions for wheat flour may result in altered product flavor or texture. Experiment with alternate flours for acceptable products, and don't be discouraged if a new product doesn't meet your standards. Try these substitutions for wheat:

Use any of the following as a thickening substitute for 1 tablespoon wheat flour:

> 1½ teaspoons cornstarch
>
> 1½ teaspoons potato starch*
>
> 1½ teaspoons arrowroot starch*
>
> 1½ teaspoons white, brown, or sweet rice flour*
>
> 2 teaspoons quick-cooking tapioca*

Use any of the following as a baking substitute for 1 cup wheat flour:

> 1 cup barley flour
>
> 1 cup corn flour*
>
> ¾ cup plain cornmeal, coarse*
>
> 1 scant cup plain cornmeal, fine*
>
> ⅝ cup potato starch flour*
>
> ¾ cup rice flour*
>
> 1¼ cup rye flour
>
> 1 cup rye meal
>
> 1⅓ cups ground rolled oats

Corn

Check food labels and products for the following foods, which indicate the presence of corn protein. Check with your physician and RD before eliminating all sources of corn from your diet.

---

* gluten-free products

fresh, canned, or creamed corn	baking powder (unless corn-free)	dextrose
		fructose
hominy or corn grits	corn syrup	lactic acid
maize	cornstarch	alcohol
cornmeal	modified food starch	vegetable gum
popcorn	dextrin	sorbitol
corn flour	maltodextrins	vinegar
corn sugar		

Substitutions and Dietary Management

Corn products are found in many foods, drugs, and even hygiene aids. Cornmeal is used to dust baking pans and containers and will adhere to baked products, such as French bread and English muffins. Mexican foods commonly contain corn in tortillas, chips, tamales, and other dishes. Syrups for canned fruits may contain corn. Baking powders and luncheon meat products should be checked for corn.

Alternatives

Corn oil is a pure product that does not contain the corn protein; it is acceptable for use by the corn-allergic individual. Corn-free baking powder is available for your baking needs. Other sugars such as honey, cane sugar, and maple syrup may substitute for corn syrup. Home cooking is the best alternative for the frustrated shopper trying to avoid corn-containing foods. Label reading is imperative for a corn-free diet.

Soy, Soy Products

Soy (or soybean) is a member of the legume family. Other members of the legume family include peas and beans (lentil, kidney, navy, pinto), licorice, and peanuts. Soy protein is nutritious, low in cost, and adaptive in many products, but it can be a source of allergic responses in many individuals. The potential for reactions to soy increases as the extensive use of this food in products increases.

Soy-derived "milk" is usually recommended for those with cow's milk allergy, although a casein hydrolysate formula may be recommended for the estimated 15% to 50% of infants allergic to cow's milk protein who are also allergic to soy protein.

Many commercial bakery goods and ice cream products contain soy. Cake and pancake mixes, meat substitutes such as imitation bacon bits and cholesterol-free breakfast foods, and canned condensed soups may contain soy. Pure soy oil, on the other hand, is considered nonallergenic and does not contain soy protein.

Check food labels and products for the following ingredients, which indicate soy. Consult your physician and RD before eliminating all sources of soy from your diet.

soy	soy sauce	tempeh
lecithin	soy miso	textured vegetable protein
tofu	modified food starch	
soybean flour		

Check packaged meats that use soy protein as an extender and ask about hamburger ingredients at your favorite fast-food restaurant. Soy is also used in school-lunch programs and other programs. Canned fish products may contain soy oil.

Nuts, Peanuts

Peanuts are a member of the legume family, unlike other nuts. Peanuts contain several substances that cause allergic reactions. Like soy, pure peanut oil is nonallergenic and can be used by allergic individuals.

Peanut allergy can be severe, and minute amounts of ingested peanuts may cause anaphylactic reactions. Careful label reading eliminates many packaged foods. The terms *nuts* or *nut meats* may indicate the use of peanut products. Bakery products may be suspect and cross-contamination may occur with non-peanut-containing products. Peanuts are often hidden in foods; some unusual examples of peanut-containing food mixtures include chicken salad and chili.

Some other common nuts causing allergic reactions include macadamias, cashews, hazelnuts (filberts), walnuts, pecans, almonds, and pistachios. Nuts are often hidden in breads, cereals, ice cream, candy, baked goods, salads, and vegetarian dishes.

Egg

Allergy to egg is relatively common in young children. Both egg white and egg yolk may cause allergies, although more reactions appear to be due to egg whites. Check food labels and products for the following ingredients, which indicate the presence of egg. Check with your physician and RD before eliminating all sources of egg from your diet and for adequate substitutes.

powdered or dried egg	ovalbumin	livetin
	ovomucin	ovoglobulin egg alubmin
dried egg yolk	ovomucoid	
egg white	vitellin	globulin
albumin	ovovitellin	

Substitutions and Dietary Management

Foods that may contain egg include mayonnaise products, desserts and baked products such as muffins and biscuits, batter-fried foods, and frozen foods. Other food categories containing egg include some pastas, such as egg noodles, pancake mixes, and vegetable dishes such as potato pancakes. Avoid products that are breaded or use sauces, such as custard sauce or hollandaise sauce, because eggs are a common ingredient. Some commercially prepared desserts may be egg-free.

Food Substitutes

Commercial egg substitutes are available but label reading is imperative; many low-cholesterol egg substitute products contain egg white. Check mayonnaise-substitute products for egg content. The fat substitute Simplesse also contains egg protein. Vaccine use should be discussed with your physician because vaccines such as MMR vaccine are commonly based on egg.

Baking

Xanthan gum, a substitute for gluten in yeast breads, can be used in baked goods, and water or vinegar can be used in place of eggs in some recipes. Xanthan gum can be purchased from some health food stores, some celiac groups, or food companies (see Ener-G-Foods, Inc, on p 19). Extra baking powder, oil, cornstarch, flour, or unflavored gelatin can be used in some products with good results.

Fish, Shellfish

Shellfish, which are known to cause severe reactions, include crustacea and mollusks. The crustacea family includes shrimp, lobster, prawn, crab, and crawfish (or crayfish). The mollusk family includes clams, oysters, scallops, mussels, and geoducks. Individuals allergic to one kind of shellfish may be allergic to others in the same family.

Reactions to fish are often immediate. Cooking does not change the reaction. Very sensitive individuals react to small particles of fish and even steam from cooked fish. Fish-allergic people usually must avoid all fish, although some people can tolerate freshwater fish but not saltwater fish, and vice versa. Surimi, a fish product used to make imitation crab, lobster, and shrimp, and some processed meat products should be avoided by fish-allergic people.

Fruits, Vegetables

Some citrus fruits cause diaper rash and a facial flush. Ripe foods such as tomatoes are more allergenic than unripe foods. Fortunately, these reactions tend to be outgrown as children age. Some fruits and vegetables are associated with pollen allergens. For instance, apple and cherry allergy is related to birch pollen allergy. These reactions have been called an "oral allergy syndrome."

Avoidance of citrus fruits necessitates nutritional counseling because these foods contain important nutrients. Often individuals can eat the cooked fruit or vegetable.

Other Foods

Virtually any food can cause an allergic response in sensitized individuals. Fortunately, most food-allergic individuals are not sensitive to more than two or three foods. Foods such as yeast, potatoes, beef, chicken, and spices may cause allergic reactions. Spices causing allergic reactions include paprika, mustard, coriander, cinnamon, pepper, bay leaf, and thyme. Check with your physician and RD for substitutes and a nutritionally adequate diet.

Resources

The following lists of resources and organizations may be helpful to you. Contact these organizations for further information.

Allergy and Asthma Network
Mothers of Asthmatics, Inc
2751 Prosperity Avenue
Suite 150
Fairfax, VA 22031
800/878-4403
703/641-9595
www.aanma.org

American Academy of Allergy, Asthma, & Immunology
611 East Wells Street
Milwaukee, WI 53202
800/822-2762
414/272-6071
www.aaaai.org

American College of Allergy, Asthma, & Immunology
85 West Algonquin Road
Suite 550
Arlington Heights, IL 60005
800/842-7777
http://allergy.mcg.edu

The Asthma and Allergy Foundation of America
1233 Twentieth Street NW
Suite 402
Washington, DC 20036
800/7-ASTHMA (800/727-8462)
202/466-7643
www.aafa.org

Food Allergy & Anaphylaxis Network
10400 Eaton Place
Suite 107
Fairfax, VA 22030-2208
800/929-4040
703/691-3179
www.foodallergy.org

U.S. Department of Health and Human Services
Food and Drug Administration
Center for Food Safety & Applied Nutrition
Consumer Education
200 C Street SW
Washington, DC 20204
888/723-3366
http://vm.cfsan.fda.gov/list.html

National Association of School Nurses
111 Cantril Street
Castle Rock, CO 80104
303/663-2329

References

Dong F M. *All About Food Allergy.* Philadelphia, Pa: George F Stickley Co, 1984.

The Food Allergy News Cookbook. Fairfax, Va: The Food Allergy Network, 1992.

Hagman B. *The Gluten-Free Gourmet, Living Well Without Wheat.* New York, NY: Henry Holt & Company, 1990.

Hartsook E. *Gluten Intolerance Group Cookbook.* 2nd ed. GIG, PO Box 23053, Seattle, WA 98102-0353, 1990.

Kidder B. *The Milk-Free Kitchen.* New York, NY: Henry Holt & Company, 1991.

Stern B. *The Food Book: The Complete Guide to the Most Popular Brand Name Foods in the United States.* New York, NY: Bookmark Books, Inc, 1987.

Thompson R C. Food allergies: separating fact from "hype". *FDA Consumer.* June 1986.

USDA. US Department of Health Human Services. *Cooking for People with Food Allergies.* USDA Home and Garden Bulletin No 246, 1988.

USDA. US Department of Health Human Services. *Nutrition and Your Health: Dietary Guidelines for Americans.* USDA Home and Garden Bulletin No 232, 1995.

Yoder E R. *Allergy-Free Cooking.* Reading, Mass: Addison-Wesley Publishing Co, 1987.

Zukin J. *Dairy-Free Cookbook.* Rocklin, Calif: Prima Publishing & Communications, 1989.

Zukin J. *Raising Your Child Without Milk.* Rocklin, Calif: Prima Publishing, 1996.

Special Products

Arrowhead Mills, Inc
PO Box 2059
Hereford, TX 78045
806/364-0730

Bob's Red Mill Natural Foods, Inc
5209 Southeast International Way
Milwaukie, OR 97222
800/349-2173
503/654-3215
www.bobsredmill.com

Ener-G Foods, Inc
5960 1st Avenue South
Seattle, WA 98124-5787
800/331-5222
www.ener-g.com

Hain Celestial Group
50 Charles Lindbergh Blvd.
Uniondale, NY 11553
516/237-6200
www.hain-celestial.com

Hershey Food Corporation
Allergy Information Team
PO Box 815
Hershey, PA 17033-0815
717/534-7500
www.hersheys.com

King Arthur Flour Company, Inc
135 Route 5 South
Norwich, VT 05055
800/827-6836
www.kingarthurflour.com

Kingsmill Foods Company, Ltd
1399 Kennedy Road, # 17
Scarborough, Ontario M1P1L6 Canada
416/755-1124
www.kingsmillfoods.com

Loma Linda Market & Nutrition Center
11161 Anderson Street
Loma Linda, CA 92350
909/558-4565

Lundberg Family Farms
5370 Church Street
PO Box 369
Richvale, CA 95974-0369
530/882-4551
www.lundberg.com

McNeil Consumer Health Care
7050 Camp Hill Road
Fort Washington, PA 19034
Lactaid Line
800/522-8243

Mead Johnson and Company
2400 West Lloyd Expressway
Evansville, IN 47721
812/429-5000
www.meadjohnson.com

Miss Roben's, Inc
91 Western Maryland Parkway
Suite 7
Hagerstown, MD 21740
800/891-0083
301/665-9580
www.missroben.com

Novartis Nutrition
5320 West 23rd St
St. Louis Park, MN 55416-1657
800/333-3785
612/925-2100
www.resourceathome.com

Pacific Foods of Oregon, Inc
19480 Southwest 97th Avenue
Tualatin, Oregon 97062
503/692-9666
www.pacificfoods.com

Red Mill Farms, Inc
7831 Woodmont Avenue, #190
Bethesda, MD 20814
718/384-2150
www.redmillfarms.com

Rich Products Corporation
One Robert Rich Way
Buffalo, NY 14213
716/878-8000
www.richs.com

Ross Laboratories
625 Cleveland Avenue
Columbus, OH 43216
614/624-7677
www.ross.com

R.W. Knudsen/Smuckers
PO Box 369, Speedway Avenue
Chico, CA 95927
530/899-5000
www.knudsenjuices.com

Tad Enterprises
9356 Pleasant
Tinley Park, IL 60477
800/438-6153
708/429-2101
www.tadenterprises.com

Recipes

The following recipes are milk-, egg-, wheat-, or corn-free where noted. These recipes are designed for easy preparation. Customize the recipes with the following guidelines:

- Select water-pack canned fruits instead of fruits packed in syrup to cut calories.
- Reduce or omit salt for lower-sodium products.
- Use fresh foods instead of canned foods to reduce sodium.
- Omit nuts for lower fat.
- Choose nonfat or low-fat milk in recipes calling for "milk" for lower fat.
- Use soft-tub margarine products instead of cube butter for less fat and cholesterol.
- In recipes with whole eggs, substitute 2 egg whites for each egg for less fat and cholesterol.

Diet analysis performed with Nutritionist III, version 6.0, N-Squared Computing Analytic Software, Salem, OR 97302.

Pumpkin Bread

2 loaves, 12 slices each

½ cup salad oil
1 cup sugar
1 cup firmly packed brown sugar
2 cups (1 pound) canned pumpkin
1 teaspoon vanilla
2½ cups flour
2 teaspoons baking soda
2 teaspoons pumpkin pie spice (or spice as tolerated)
1 teaspoon salt
½ cup chopped dates
½ cup chopped nuts (if tolerated)

No corn
egg
milk
soy

1. Preheat oven to 350°F.

2. Grease two 9" × 5" loaf pans.

3. Combine oil, sugars, pumpkin, and vanilla in mixing bowl. Beat well.

4. Add sifted dry ingredients. Mix just until all dry ingredients are moistened. Fold in dates and nuts.

5. Pour batter into pans and bake 1 hour. Bread may be glazed with 1 cup sifted confectioners' sugar mixed with 2 tablespoons hot water if desired.

Each slice provides:

165 Calories   30 g Carbohydrates
1 g Protein   161 mg Sodium
5 g Fat   0 mg Cholesterol

Rye Bread

2 loaves, 12 slices each

6 cups 100% rye flour
1 tablespoon salt
2 packages dry yeast
½ cup instant mashed potatoes
2 cups hot tap water
½ cup molasses (if not tolerated, substitute sugar)
¼ cup salad oil

No corn
egg
milk
soy
wheat

1. In large mixer bowl, thoroughly mix 2 cups flour with salt and undissolved yeast.

2. Add instant mashed potatoes to hot water. Whip lightly with fork.

3. Combine liquids (molasses and oil) and potato and water mixture. Add to dry ingredients.

4. Beat 2 minutes at medium speed of mixer, scraping bowl occasionally.

5. Add 2 cups flour. Beat at high speed 2 minutes, scraping bowl occasionally.

6. Stir in remaining 2 cups flour (or enough to make a stiff dough).

7. Sprinkle bread board with rye flour. Turn dough out and knead until smooth and elastic (8 to 10 minutes).

8. Place dough in greased bowl; cover and let rise in warm place until double in bulk (1½ to 2 hours).

9. Grease two 9" × 5" loaf pans.

10. Punch down dough and shape into 2 loaves. Cover and let rise until double in bulk (30 to 45 minutes).

11. Preheat oven to 350°F.

12. Bake 40 minutes or until loaves sound hollow when tapped lightly.

Each slice provides:

140	Calories	27 g	Carbohydrate
3 g	Protein	299 mg	Sodium
3 g	Fat	0 mg	Cholesterol

White Bread

2 loaves, 12 slices each

7 cups flour
2 packages dry yeast
3 tablespoons sugar
1 tablespoon salt
¼ cup instant mashed potatoes
2 cups very hot tap water
¼ cup margarine

No corn
egg
milk
soy

1. Combine thoroughly in mixer bowl 2 cups flour, dry yeast, sugar, and salt.

2. Mix instant potatoes with hot water and margarine. Add to dry ingredients. Beat for 2 minutes at medium speed, scraping bowl.

3. Add 2 cups flour. Beat on high speed for another 2 minutes. Stir in remaining flour with a spoon.

4. Turn out on floured board; knead until smooth and elastic (8 to 10 minutes).

5. Place in greased bowl, cover and let rise in warm place until doubled in bulk (1 hour). Punch dough down.

6. Turn out on floured board. Cover and let rise 15 minutes.

7. Grease two 9" × 5" loaf pans.

8. Divide dough in half and shape into 2 loaves. Place in pans. Cover and let rise until double in bulk (1 hour).

9. Preheat oven to 400°F.

10. Bake 25 to 30 minutes or until loaf sounds hollow when tapped lightly with finger.

Each slice provides:

160	Calories	30 g	Carbohydrate
4 g	Protein	305 mg	Sodium
2 g	Fat	0 mg	Cholesterol

Oatmeal Crackers

4 dozen

4	cups oatmeal
½	cup salad oil
2	tablespoons sugar
1	teaspoon salt
¾	cup lukewarm water

No corn
egg
milk
soy
wheat

1. Preheat oven to 325°F.

2. Thoroughly combine oatmeal and salad oil. Mix in sugar and salt.

3. Add water and mix well. Dough will be slightly sticky.

4. Divide dough into 2 parts. Roll each part to ⅛" thickness between 2 sheets of foil.

5. Transfer foil and dough to baking sheet. Peel off top sheet of foil and cut dough into squares. Sprinkle with salt if desired.

6. Bake 15 minutes until lightly browned.

Each cracker provides:

75	Calories	27 g	Carbohydrate
7 g	Protein	145 mg	Sodium
9 g	Fat	0 mg	Cholesterol

Rice and Barley Muffins

6 muffins

⅓	cup rice flour
⅔	cup barley flour
3	teaspoons baking powder
2	tablespoons sugar
¼	teaspoon salt
¾	cup milk
1	tablespoon margarine, melted

No egg
soy
wheat

1. Preheat oven to 375°F.

2. Grease muffin pans (2½" × 1¼").

3. Mix and sift dry ingredients together.

4. Add milk and melted margarine. Stir only enough to combine.

5. Fill muffin pans two-thirds full.

6. Bake 20 minutes until lightly browned.

From *All About Food Allergy* by Faye M Dong. Reprinted with permission from George F Stickley Co.

Banana Pancakes   *10 pancakes*

. . . .

1⅓   cups oat flour

1½   teaspoons corn-free baking powder

1   tablespoon granulated sugar

¼   teaspoon cinnamon
    Pinch of cloves

1   cup single-strength soy milk OR nondairy
    creamer (diluted ⅔ cup creamer + ⅓ cup water)

2   tablespoons melted margarine

1   egg, beaten

1   medium-size banana

No corn
    milk
    wheat

Stir together flour, baking powder, sugar, cinnamon, and cloves. Add soy milk or nondairy creamer, melted margarine, and egg; mix well. If batter is too thick, add a little more milk or creamer. Thinly slice the banana and fold into batter. Bake on hot griddle. Serve with allowed syrup or fresh fruit in its own juice.

Each pancake provides:
130	Calories	18 g	Carbohydrate
5 g	Protein	90 mg	Sodium
5 g	Fat	21 mg	Cholesterol

From *All About Food Allergy* by Faye M Dong. Reprinted with permission from George F Stickley Co.

Basic Pancakes or Waffles

8 servings

2 cups rice flour
1 tablespoon sugar
4 teaspoons baking powder
1 teaspoon salt
4 egg whites
1½ cups low-fat or nonfat milk
¼ cup salad oil

No soy
wheat

1. Sift together dry ingredients

2. Beat together egg whites, milk, and oil. Add to dry ingredients, mixing just until dry ingredients are moistened.

3. Bake on hot, greased griddle or waffle iron.

> *Variations:* Fold in ⅓ cup of any of the following if tolerated: diced ham, bits of crisp bacon, raisins, chopped dates, slivered dried apricots, finely diced raw apple, or drained and chopped cooked prunes.
>
> Shortcake: Fold stiffly beaten egg whites into batter. Bake on waffle iron. Serve with sweetened berries or fruit.

Each serving provides:

235	Calories	36 g	Carbohydrate
6 g	Protein	482 mg	Sodium
7 g	Fat	1 mg	Cholesterol

Orange Rolls

Makes 18 rolls

Dough:

¼ cup margarine
½ teaspoon salt
¼ cup granulated sugar
1 cup milk, scalded and cooled to lukewarm
1 package active dry yeast
¼ cup warm water
1 teaspoon egg substitute (egg-free) + 2 tablespoons water (thoroughly mixed together)
4 cups all-purpose white wheat flour (approximately): sift before measuring
Margarine, softened, 1 tablespoon

No corn
egg
soy

Filling:

½ cup softened margarine
⅓ cup granulated sugar
Grated peel of 2 medium-size oranges

Put the margarine, salt, and sugar in a large bowl. Add the luke-warm milk and stir until the dry ingredients are dissolved. Soften the yeast in the warm water and add it, along with the beaten egg, to the milk mixture. Stir in 3½ cups of the flour, 1 cup at a time, beating until blended. Scrape the dough from the sides of the bowl, making a large ball of dough, and brush the top of the dough and the sides of the bowl with the softened margarine. Cover with waxed paper and a damp cloth. Let rise in a warm place for about 2 hours, or until almost doubled in bulk. Turn out onto a well-floured board and knead lightly, adding flour until the dough is no longer sticky (do not use more than ¼ to ½ cup flour on the board).

Cream together the filling ingredients until smooth. Roll out the dough to a rectangle about ¼" thick. Spread the filling mixture evenly over the dough. Roll the dough up jelly-roll fashion and then chill in the refrigerator for at least an hour. With a very sharp knife, cut chilled dough into 1" slices and place 1" apart on greased baking sheets. Let rise in a warm place until almost doubled in size. Bake at 425°F for 10 to 14 minutes. Remove from baking sheet immediately with a spatula and place on plates (if rolls are going to be served right away) or on cooling racks (if rolls are to be served later).

If the rolls are going to be served later, reheat briefly in the oven at 350°F.

Each roll provides:

195	Calories	26 g	Carbohydrate
3 g	Protein	177 mg	Sodium
8 g	Fat	0 g	Cholesterol

From *All About Food Allergy* by Faye M Dong. Reprinted with permission from George F Stickley Co.

Hearty Ham Casserole

6 servings

2   tablespoons milk-free margarine
2   teaspoons rice flour
2½   cups single-strength soy milk
      Salt and pepper to taste
2   garlic cloves, minced
½   white onion, minced
      Safflower oil
4   potatoes, pared and thinly sliced
1   piece, approximately 4" × 6", yellow squash (butternut or marble), peeled and sliced like the potatoes
3   cups ham, diced or shredded
½   medium zucchini, chopped

No corn egg milk wheat

Make cream sauce by melting margarine, blending in flour, then slowly adding soy milk, stirring constantly. Season sauce with a pinch of salt and pepper to taste. Stir in garlic and onion. Pour a small amount of sauce in the bottom of a baking dish that has been greased with safflower oil. Alternate layers of potato, squash, ham, and zucchini in baking dish. Pour remainder of sauce over casserole and bake, covered, at 350°F in center of oven for about 1 hour, or until potatoes are tender.

Each serving provides:

290	Calories	36 g	Carbohydrate
24 g	Protein	950 mg	Sodium
6 g	Fat	39 mg	Cholesterol

From *All About Food Allergy* by Faye M Dong. Reprinted with permission from George F Stickley Co.

Fruit Sauce

4 servings, each ¼ cup

1   cup fruit juice (apricot, cherry, peach, grape, or pineapple)
2   tablespoons sugar
1   tablespoon cornstarch or 2 tablespoons rice flour
2   tablespoons cold water

No egg milk soy wheat

1. Heat juice and sugar to boiling.

2. Mix cornstarch or rice flour with cold water to a smooth paste.

3. Add to hot juice, stirring constantly. Cook slowly until thick and clear. May be served with fruit pudding, boiled rice, desserts, or allowed cereals.

Each serving provides:

65	Calories	16 g	Carbohydrate
0 g	Protein	1 mg	Sodium
0 g	Fat	0 mg	Cholesterol

Chiffon Cake   *12 servings*

· ·

¾   cup rice flour
¾   cup sugar
2   teaspoons baking powder
½   teaspoon salt
¼   cup salad oil
3   egg yolks
¼   cup water
1   teaspoon vanilla extract
3   egg whites
¼   teaspoon cream of tartar

No milk
soy
wheat

1. Preheat oven to 325°F.

2. Sift together dry ingredients.

3. Add oil, egg, yolks, water, and vanilla. Beat until very smooth.

4. Beat egg whites and cream of tartar until whites form very stiff peaks. Fold into egg yolk mixture.

5. Pour into ungreased 9" tube pan.

6. Bake 35 minutes or until firm to the touch. Invert pan to cool. Cool completely before removing from pan.

Variations: Coffee Chiffon: Add 2 teaspoons instant coffee to dry ingredients.

Lemon Chiffon: Substitute 1 teaspoon lemon extract for vanilla. Add 1 tablespoon fresh, grated lemon rind.

Maple Chiffon: Substitute 1 teaspoon imitation maple flavoring for vanilla.

Peppermint Chiffon: Substitute 1 teaspoon peppermint flavoring for vanilla. Add few drops red food coloring.

Each serving provides:

140	Calories	20 g	Carbohydrate
2 g	Protein	160 mg	Sodium
6 g	Fat	53 mg	Cholesterol

Eggless Chocolate Cake

8 servings

1½ cups pure all-purpose white wheat flour
1 cup granulated sugar
3 tablespoons unsweetened cocoa powder
1½ teaspoons corn-free baking powder
1 teaspoon baking soda
½ teaspoon salt
1 cup cold water
¼ cup + 1 tablespoon allowed vegetable oil (no olive oil)
1 tablespoon fresh lemon juice
1½ teaspoons vanilla extract

No corn egg soy

In a medium-size bowl, stir together flour, sugar, cocoa, baking powder, soda, and salt. Make a well in the center. Pour water, oil, lemon juice, and vanilla into well; beat until smooth (batter will be thin). Pour into greased and floured 8" square pan. Bake at 350°F for 30 to 35 minutes, until tester inserted in center comes out clean. Invert cake onto wire rack to cool.

Each serving provides:

260	Calories	43 g	Carbohydrate
3 g	Protein	297 mg	Sodium
9 g	Fat	1 mg	Cholesterol

From *All About Food Allergy* by Faye M Dong. Reprinted with permission from George F Stickley Co.

Swiss Jelly Roll

12 servings

1 recipe Chiffon Cake, mixed in bowl
1 cup crab apple jelly or jam
¼ cup confectioners' sugar

No milk soy wheat

1. Preheat oven to 350°F.

2. Line jelly roll pan (12" × 16" × 1") with waxed paper.

3. Spread batter in pan.

4. Bake 20 minutes. Invert on towel sprinkled with confectioners' sugar. Trim off crisp edges; roll up and cool.

5. When cool, unroll and spread with crab apple jelly. Reroll and sift confectioners' sugar over top.

   Variation: Substitute any other jelly of your choice.

   ### Each serving provides:

215	Calories	40 g	Carbohydrate
2 g	Protein	164 mg	Sodium
6 g	Fat	53 mg	Cholesterol

Molasses Drop Cookies *24 servings, 2 cookies each*

· ·

½ cup margarine
½ cup sugar
½ cup molasses
2 cups 100% rye flour
2 teaspoons baking powder
¼ teaspoon ground ginger
½ teaspoon nutmeg
½ cup applesauce
½ cup raisins (rinsed with hot water)

No egg
milk
soy
wheat

1. Preheat oven to 375°F.

2. Grease baking sheet.

3. Cream together margarine, sugar, and molasses.

4. Sift together dry ingredients. Add alternately with applesauce to creamed mixture. Add raisins.

5. Drop by rounded teaspoons on baking sheet.

6. Bake 10 minutes

   ### Each serving provides:

110	Calories	18 g	Carbohydrate
1 g	Protein	74 mg	Sodium
4 g	Fat	0 mg	Cholesterol

Oatmeal Lace Cookies

30 servings, 2 cookies each

1 cup margarine
1 cup firmly packed brown sugar
1 cup sugar
1 teaspoon vanilla extract
1 cup rice flour
1 teaspoon salt
4 teaspoons baking powder
¾ cup water
3 cups oatmeal
½ cup chopped nuts (if tolerated)

1. Preheat oven to 350°F.

2. Grease baking sheet.

3. Cream margarine, sugars, and vanilla.

4. Sift together rice flour, salt, and baking powder. Add dry ingredients alternately to creamed mixture with water.

5. Add oatmeal and nuts; mix well. Dough may be chilled if desired.

6. Drop by teaspoons on baking sheet.

7. Bake 10 minutes.

Each serving provides:

200	Calories	29 g	Carbohydrate
3 g	Protein	189 mg	Sodium
8 g	Fat	0 mg	Cholesterol

Lemon Pie

9" pie, 8 servings

1 cup sugar
¼ cup cornstarch or ½ cup rice flour
½ teaspoon salt
1 cup water
2 tablespoons grated lemon rind
½ cup lemon juice
2 tablespoons milk-free margarine
1 Crumb Crust (follows)

1. Mix sugar, cornstarch or rice flour, and salt together in saucepan.

2: Stir water in gradually. Cook over medium heat, stirring constantly, until mixture thickens and boils.

3. When mixture is clear, add lemon rind, juice, and margarine. Remove from heat. Chill before using.

4. Spoon into baked pie crust. Chill until serving time. May be garnished with nondairy whipped topping (check label).

Each serving provides:

280	Calories	48 g	Carbohydrate
1 g	Protein	427 mg	Sodium
11 g	Fat	0 mg	Cholesterol

Crumb Crust
9" pie, 8 servings

. . . .

1	cup crushed, crisp rice cereal
¼	cup sugar
⅓	cup milk-free margarine or shortening, melted

No egg milk wheat

1. Preheat oven to 375°F.

2. Mix cereal crumbs, sugar, and melted shortening.

3. Press firmly into bottom and sides of pie pan.

4. Bake 8 minutes until lightly browned. Crust may be refrigerated for 1 hour before filling instead of baking.

Variations: Crushed corn cereal may be used in place of rice cereal. Oatmeal may be used in place of rice cereal, but this crust must be baked.

Each serving provides:

145	Calories	18 g	Carbohydrate
1 g	Protein	259 mg	Sodium
8 g	Fat	0 mg	Cholesterol